HopeWorks Medical Diary

A Patient's Daily Log ™

by

Donna L. Hope
with
The Cunningham Family

Disclaimer

The purpose of this book is to provide ample space for individuals to keep a record of information pertaining to one's health. All questions or inquires regarding health issues should be directed to the patient's doctor(s).

This book was created for convenience, and with love and support as the primary issue based on our experience...not with the intent to be hurtful, or to cause harm. The author, Cunningham Family and/or HopeWorks are not responsible for any loss, damage or misfortune.

If you do not wish to be bound by the above, you may return this book to the publisher for a full refund.

Printed by:

Hignell Printing Limited
Winnipeg Manitoba Canada

ISBN: 0-9657195-0-2

Copyright 1996 by Donna L. Hope. All Rights Reserved Worldwide. No part of this book may be reproduced, transmitted, photocopied, altered, modified, recorded, electronic, or mechanical, including storage and retrieval systems, or otherwise, in any form or by any means without written permission from the author.

HopeWorks
Medical Diary

FOR

Name: _____

Phone: (_____) _____

Doctor: _____
_____
(_____) _____

Patient diagnosed with:

_____

Foreword

The fight against cancer is often a massive undertaking. Donna Hope and the Cunningham family have created this diary to assist the patient and family in this fight. They are particularly suited to this task, since they recently experienced a long and difficult battle themselves. They came to realize that there are very few situations where better communication does not help. The illness itself, aggressive therapies applied to the illness, and the resulting emotional turmoil, create a large opportunity for confusion. This patient's daily log should do much to overcome much of the confusion and the errors that can result from such a state.

Every aspect of the interaction between the health care team and the patient's family unit are well covered in this diary. I would encourage individuals using this diary to keep it with them on visits to the hospital or physician's office. It affords an opportunity to prepare a written list of questions which is not only efficient, but timesaving for everyone, including the health care team. In addition, there is ample space for precisely writing down the instructions given to the patient, thereby avoiding errors of communication. A glance at the activity log by members of the health care team utilizes only a fraction of the time required to obtain the same information from questioning. In short, I believe that this tool is an asset for both the patient/family unit and the health care team, and I encourage its use. The authors have learned this methodology the hard way and have graciously made it available so that others need not learn by trial and error.

Philip J. DiSaia, M.D.
The Dorothy Marsh Chair in Reproductive Biology
Director, Division of Gynecologic Oncology
Professor, Department of Obstetrics and Gynecology

There are times in the practice of medicine when physicians are privileged to not only observe, but participate in the best of our human condition. Strength and personal character are important threads of our civilization and society, but examples are few and far between, unfortunately. In adverse times, those qualities can and do prevail.

When I first met Elsa Cunningham, those qualities so eloquently described by her daughter in this book were obvious within the first ten minutes of a conversation. Sadly, so were the findings of adversity, a potentially large cancer. In the best tradition of human experience. Elsa took the news as anyone reading this book would. She was scared. Shortly her strength of character and positive outlook began to emerge, along with the support of her family which was considerable. Elsa faced her treatment determined to continue her life's forward view, with goals of continuing to dance and remain close to her family. She fought the battle in order to smile, but what emerged was much more than that. As I spoke from time to time with her family, I could understand how they were strengthened by this positive approach. We all were comforted that in the time she had left on earth she helped push those around her to higher levels than they were before.

One magnificent example of the higher levels of achievement is this book for patients and families facing similar circumstances. Not only will this book give helpful organization for any patient with cancer, but also other chronic, time and treatment intensive disease or condition. The organization tips for families and patients will save time, effort and, consequently no doubt, unnecessary sorrow and grief. In the process of using this book, the readers will receive the largest benefit of easily understanding the meaning of a positive attitude. Any physician could tell you it does make a difference in outcome, especially in quality of life.

Not only did Elsa and her family refuse to give up and quit; not only did Elsa and her family extract so much for themselves with this positive loving attitude; but also they captured this spirit and now share it with others. That is the main point of this book, and it is easy to feel by reading. In my humble opinion, many will benefit from this family's strength in the face of adversity.

Edwin B. Shackeroff, M.D., F.A.C.O.G.
Los Alamitos, California

What People Are Saying About
HopeWorks Medical Diary...A Patient's Daily Log

"Finally! An educational and constructive project for the non-medically trained family member or loved one. Maintaining this journal will help relieve the gnawing feeling of helplessness felt by anyone who has lost a loved one due to a protracted illness. It will also be an excellent reference for any other family members who may endure similar afflictions in the future."
— Kathleen Dyer, daughter of cancer patient Carolyn Beld 1945 - 1991.

"...a terrific blend of your own experience and an invitation to others to add their own ideas or adapt this resource to meet their own unique needs."
— Jo Michelle Beld, Ph.D.

"The Information Section is wonderful. So often patients do not remember to bring the information with them because they are overwhelmed with everything. This is one less thing they have to worry about."
— Andree Liebel, R.N.

"...relevant to the total personal care of the patient, rather than just their medical needs."
— Linda Lubking, Financial Counselor S.C.M.C. CNA, HHA Activities Director

"Sections are easily explained...you have done a remarkable job in putting this helpful dairy together. Good job! Well done!"
— Patricia A. Greenfield, R.N.

"An invaluable resource tool to be used as you assist in the care of someone dear to you as they face some of the most difficult days of their lives. It allows you and the patient to be prepared at all times with the immediate, necessary information for successful care and decision-making. This would be extremely useful for Paramedic and emergency room teams should the situation occur."
— Denise Mascarella, daughter of cancer patient, Dennis Carlson 1930-1990

PREFACE

Charting the course of Mom's illness on a daily basis turned into *The HopeWorks Medical Diary*. Each section serves a particular purpose, making it possible to use the journal as a workbook or daily log.

The purpose of this book is to help people with any type of serious or terminal illness to record daily information regarding their health. The records will benefit doctors, caregivers and--most importantly--the patient by keeping track of daily activities, medications, appointments and anything else to help ease stress in an unsettling and frustrating time in his/her life.

During our personal experiences we were able to answer questions and also to refer back to certain situations. The doctor asked for important details regarding something Mom could or could not tolerate, concerning: chemotherapy, implants, radiation, medicines, pain relievers...etc. With the help of this book, we were able to answer the questions.

We had no idea what the doctor might need. Documenting everything helped provide the necessary information and guided us through this puzzling time, making it well worth the effort. The doctors were very pleased with the written correspondence we provided at each office visit.

Not only did we apprise ourselves with the written data we had, we became well educated with the type of illness Mom had. The more we filled in the blanks...the more questions we asked...the more knowledge we gained. This allowed us to communicate, understand, and clearly respond to everyone medically involved with our Mom's declining health.

This book will prove most valuable when used daily. Take the journal with you when you go for an appointment; to the hospital; at home; or any time you need to record information or refer back to prior data. You will be amazed at the handiness of this book, and how often you will use it.

Dedication

This Medical Diary is dedicated to our wonderful mother, Elsa Mae Cunningham.

We love you deeply.

This book is a tribute to you.

Your children and grandchildren: Ronda, Donna, Roger, Matt and Marshall.

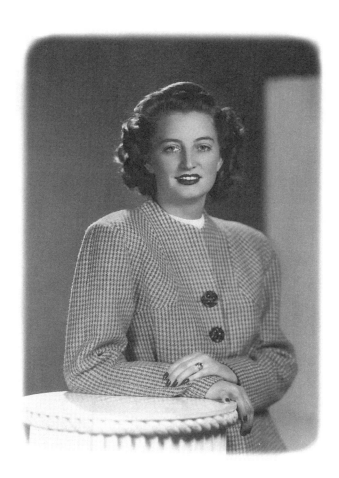

Elsa M. Cunningham

A Special Thanks

To Doctors: Shackeroff, DiSaia, Monk, Brewer, Hess, Bernstein, and to: Terry, Flo, Mouna: her Pharmacist...for their constant care and concern for our dear Mother.

Acknowledgments

A heartfelt thanks to Dad, family and friends for the support, compassion, phone calls, visits and being available when we needed you. Your love and devotion carried us through very difficult times.

We would like to express our gratitude to our editor, Shirl Thomas for her encouragement in helping to make this book a reality.

The Cunningham Family

Our family life is well remembered. Dad, Mom, three kids and pets, all along the way. Dad...always the quiet analytical one; Mom...outgoing, witty, funny--and she loved to entertain. All family get-togethers and holiday gatherings were held at our home...a perfect place for every occasion with a large yard to play volleyball and basketball games, and to jump up and down on our tractor tire inner tube. We'd gather for most any reason to play games and laugh until we fell off our chairs.

Years passed and we established our own lives. Always a close family, we called our parents and each other daily, to report in. We continued to find excuses for all of us to gather together with our families and friends, so we could laugh--sometimes, until the tears rolled down our faces.

As we kids reached our forties, Mom and Dad turned seventy. In addition to keeping busy with home, work, church and kids--together, they square danced, round danced, fished, and did a fantastic jiggerbug. Dad enjoys his bridge club, golfing, baseball, and the Begonia club. Mom had her favorites too, like: clogging, bingo, bowling, walking, card parties, traveling, Senior Citizen groups, McDonnell Douglas Retirees Luncheon Club, 1984 Olympics volunteer, and she dearly loved volunteering at the Orange County Fairgrounds.

Over time, we became aware that Mom did not feel healthy enough to continue normal activities. Something was wrong. She became less active. The reason for her unexplainable pain was discovered. Mom had a cyst and needed a hysterectomy, which revealed the cyst was malignant, and next, came radiation and implants. Mom had a fast moving cancer that could reappear anywhere, anytime.

One year later, a second tumor was discovered in her pelvic area. Growing to the point where something needed to be done, the doctors removed what they could, after chemotherapy no longer had an impact. Unfortunately, they couldn't get all the cancer. Soon, Mom was back in the hospital, uncomfortable and dying. All through her battle we prayed for her to live, and for great insight to come to the doctors, and nurses. The doctors, interns and staff were wonderful. They counseled showing kindness, compassion, patience, giving Mother (and us) their undivided attention.

As time went by, it became apparent that the Lord's will was taking our Mother in a different direction. Seeing Mom suffer so badly, we kids began to pray for the Lord to take her home. It was most difficult and emotionally upsetting to face the fact that we wouldn't have Mom much longer, and that she would never spend another Christmas with us.

We couldn't imagine life without her. She was so active, vivacious, positive, and turned ordinary smiles into chuckles or laughter. Nothing stopped her, an elegant lady who loved life.

Although death was not the miracle we prayed for, it was the miracle that God chose. He gave us the privilege to return the care that Mom always gave us...back to her. We stayed by Mom's side constantly, at home and in the hospital, and took her to most all of her appointments, and when we couldn't, a relative or close friend did. We did everything we could for her and appreciated the opportunity to do so.

Days and weeks went by. We agreed not to tell Mom everything the doctors related, nor did she want to know. She had hopes of recovering and returning to an active life. Hope gave her something to look forward to each new day. It gave her a reason to wake up and look out the window to see the sun shining, or watch the birds. The drugs didn't allow her to remember much, anyway.

Mom seemed comfortable at home. We sat beside her and tried to carry on normal, everyday conversations as she lay in bed, asleep. We reminisced, and tears filled our eyes and hearts. We have always been a family who often repeats, "I Love You." Losing Mom seemed to give a new and greater meaning to those words.

Mom was a "Classy Lady." She was physically pretty, meticulous, dressed nicely and looked radiant in her favorite color...red. Mom never complained, and always looked at the bright side of every situation. Besides being a wonderful lady, she was a terrific secretary...with a gift of organization. It became difficult for her to deal with a awful situation...taking control without her permission!

As Mom's body deteriorated she could no longer do much for herself. Even moving from one side to another became difficult and frustrating. Mom cried a lot; and so did we.

During her final stage, she tried to be a frisky fighter, but her witty personality seemed to disappear...too weak, too worn out to fight. For two long years we watched Mom lose her health and her strength. We watched a very elegant lady give in to the ugliness of cancer. It was hard to see a woman of perfection - highly respected and admired by her family and peers--die. From the beginning, at her request, there would be no visitors at the hospital nor at home. She didn't ever want anyone to see what this disease had done to her. She felt so embarrassed, but could do nothing to stop it.

She prayed. We prayed. She slept. We watched. She suffered. We waited.

The time came for all of us to let go...time to tell Mom we'd be all right. She fought death...she needed to hear that we would be OK.

On Tuesday, April 22nd we were all in her bedroom. It was evident that a new adventure for Mom was only hours to minutes away. We sat on the bed, as she lay there sleeping. Her heart worked hard to keep up. We quietly reminisced, once more, about our growing up and all the wonderful memories she gave us. We read the Bible to her and we prayed. Early Wednesday, at 1:20 a.m., Mom's breathing became shallow and faint. We knelt down beside her with our hands on her heart and said:

"It's time to go with the angels. It's okay. We love you, and we'll miss you. You'll get to walk again. You'll see so many new things...so many new colors. You will even get to see what God and Jesus really look like! And all of your loved ones and friends who are already there will be waiting to greet you. So, let go of us. We release you. We ALL love you. Good-bye Mom. The angels are here now; go with them."

As she took her last breath, we held hands and prayed. Immediately, we felt her spirit in the room. Looking up, we talked to her, and it comforted us in knowing she will always be a part of our lives.

Now Mom is free from pain...free from being motionless. She won't remember the pain, only the love.

Our family shared love and grief. As the days pass we still seem to be exhausted. Emotionally, we still cry. Mentally, she's all we think about. Physically, we are simply worn-out. Although life is lonely without her, we have no regrets. Mom never knew a day without our devoted love, care, concern and support. The importance of family unity is as beautiful and unexplainable as the word love. It is such a rewarding feeling to comfort and encourage one another.

Mom's Memorial Service was a credit to her. The lobby of the church was beautifully adorned with memories of Elsa: Mom, Relative and Friend. Pictures of her from birth ..., filled tables from one end to the other. Each picture captured the joy, laughter, activities, and experience of each stage in her life. Every individual could relate to how they fit in.

er wedding dress hung from the balcony. Pretty square-dance skirts she had sewn from her antique sewing machine (that could only sew a straight stitch) hung beside the specially designed family reunion shirt along with her 1984 Olympics volunteer outfit and relics. Get well and other greeting cards filled baskets by the door. Sad faces turned to smiles as they were surrounded with family and friends reminiscing about their own personal friendships with a great lady.

Her telephone is still connected and the answering machine is on, so we can call to hear her heartwarming voice. This helps to fill the emptiness and comforts us.

The name, Elsa, fit her well. It means, Noble: great, and dignified. Mom suffered badly with cancer, but she died with dignity.

We thank God for having blessed us with our Mom. She might have thought some of the things she did for us went unnoticed; but we noticed. She had a greater and more powerful influence on us than she could ever know. We will always hold a special place for her in our hearts, and we will honor her, forever. In countless ways she shared her warmth, caring and understanding. Mom's cheerfulness enriched us. Our lives became a colorful rainbow because of the beautiful person she was.

Thank you for the memories, Mom. We love you,   Ronda, Donna and Roger

How To Use This Book

The *HopeWorks Medical Diary* is laid out in sections rather than chapters because it is designed for journalizing. It will assist in maintaining all pertinent information. Each section was devised to serve a particular purpose, making it possible to use the journal as a workbook or daily log. Anyone should be able to pick up this book and access what is happening.

There are **fourteen Sections**:

Section 1...The **Appointment Calendar**: Use this to keep track of scheduled appointments of anything you want to remember on a specific day.

Section 2...The **Daily Health Chart** is for keeping track of the details regarding an ailing individual's well being, or physical activities for each day. It is set up as a weekly schedule with space for the day and time, and to fill in the appropriate description, such as: temperature; weight; appetite; "toileting"; exercises, or any type of detailed information regarding a patient's daily existence.

Section 3...The **Daily Medication Log**: List patient's medication and the time taken. Heavily medicated patients lose track easily. This section helps to prevent the patient from taking too many doses and keeps them right on target for when the next time medication should be administered. In most cases, patients are on more than one strong drug or narcotic at a time. This is the best way to keep a patient safe from harming themselves with too much medication taken accidentally and/or to close together.

Many people's illnesses require more than one medicine, whether taken jointly or periodically. Most medications can have a side effect. Listing particular problems and/or successful remedies in **Section 4**, the **Medicine Section** makes it possible to refer back in order to clarify anything regarding the different types, doses and patient's reactions. **Section 5...Questions for the Doctor** will house the list of things you want to remember to ask, for example: "What is going to happen?" "When...?" "How long does it take?" ... all of the when's, what's, where's, why and how's. This is a perfect place to jot down those questions for in-between visits and phone calls. Recording the various types of **Tests and Results,** in **Section 6** will be useful to both patient and doctor. The type, reason, and the result of test(s) will be conveniently listed here for future reference.

Section 7 is based on the **Surgery/Hospital Stay**. Although most individuals go through this ordeal only once or twice, others may require devising a track record for reoccurring visits. Often many illnesses lead to constant research for supplies and/or support groups--both physical and mental. Patients may be referred by their doctors or by "word of mouth." Writing down these names and places in **Referrals...Section 8**, can save hours on this time consuming project. The **Helpful Hints...Section 9**, is our family favorite. Over the two year period, it became increasingly difficult for Mother to accomplish daily tasks. With her help, we developed shortcuts that made life bearable. Everyone who has an illness can find helpful shortcuts. Mom greatly benefited as we utilized the helpful hints and quickly made any necessary changes in the way we approached feeding, bathing, moving her, and in any other care giving process.

Mom kept a Diary to document her feelings, pains reactions and struggles. **Section 10** is reserved for use as a Personal Diary. Use as you would any diary.

Mom needed to communicate in order to detail things to be done. The information filed in **Section 11**, the **Notes** section, replaces those pieces of paper that could otherwise get lost in the shuffle. From the simplest item to remember, such as--what to pick up at the grocery store, to...the more important--what to take to the hospital. Writing things down became great reminders.

At times there will be a need for **Section 12...Messages**. Rather than risk waking the patient or causing confusion during a care giver's shift change, leaving messages helps the next person and is a good way to communicate between each other without disturbing the patient. This section is reserved for writing down questions, comments, notes for follow-up and any other items of importance, making it easy for the next caregiver to take over and pick up where the previous caregiver left off. This also applies when the patient is changing location for any reason.

Section 13...Miscellaneous: A place to store such items as: copies of maps; prescriptions; any paperwork or receipts; and the hospital's layout showing where to go for tests--what floor, and what hospital wing. This very important grouping is efficiently accessible, and kept altogether in one place.

Section 14—final section--a suggestion sheet has been provided for any comments you may have, in addition to your original helpful hints. Because this journal will be updated annually, any suggestions for making the journal even better will be appreciated.

Having the following items available will greatly facilitate using this book.

Three ring binder - 1 to 1 1/2" depth.

Self adhesive tabs...for easy access to individual sections.

Plastic zippered pocket pouch and/or file folder with pockets

for miscellaneous items, including:

business cards
directions/maps
information pamphlets
instructions
paperwork
parking passes
pencils
pens
prescriptions
receipts
signed documents

Keep extra copies in binder, if needed:

Birth Certificate
Blood Donor Card
Drivers License
Health Care Power of Attorney
(Living Will)
Insurance Information
Social Security Card

Our hearts are with you as you journey through HopeWorks Medical Diary.

The Cunningham Family

Table of Contents

Table of Contents

Personal Information

Telephone Numbers and Addresses

Appointment Calendar...*Section 1 / Page 25*
    A convenient way to schedule appointments for Doctors, Specialists, Chemotherapy, Physical Therapy, etc.

Daily Health Chart..*Section 2 / Page 43*
    A simple health record kept on a daily basis.

Daily Medication Log...*Section 3 / Page 101*
    An easy way to record the name and type of medication, dosage, and to keep track of the day and time taken.

Medicine..*Section 4 / Page 159*
    In this section you can record detailed information regarding why certain medicines were prescribed for you.

Questions for the Doctor(s)..*Section 5 / Page 177*
    Sometimes it is difficult to remember all the necessary things to discuss with the doctor; this section makes it a lot easier.

Tests and Results..*Section 6 / Page 187*
    Information and assessments of tests are recorded here for the convenience of patient and doctor(s).

Surgery/Hospital Stay..................................... *Section 7 / Page 201*
> Dates and information.

Referrals.. *Section 8 / Page 215*
> A great way to remember support and therapy groups, where to purchase supplies, and miscellaneous.

Helpful Hints... *Section 9 / Page 229*
> Ideas, advice, and suggestions of benefit during illness or recovery.

Personal Diary.. *Section 10 / Page 245*
> Keeping a journal by day, week or month is a valuable reference tool.

Notes.. *Section 11 / Page 309*
> Taking notes will help in keeping clear details and instructions.

Messages... *Section 12 / Page 323*
> Writing messages is a good way for the patient and/or caregivers to communicate with each other.

Miscellaneous.. *Section 13 / Page 347*
> This section is provided to keep copies of signed documents, receipts, maps or directions to appointment locations, etc.

Comments and Suggestions............................ *Section 14 / Page 355*
> A space is provided for comments and suggestions. All are most welcome.

Order Form...*Page 359*

Personal Information

Personal Information

Copies of pertinent information allow easier access for various sources, such as doctors, clinics, etc. This is especially helpful when entering the hospital emergency room.

For example:

- Birth Certificate
- Blood Donor Card
- Drivers License
- Health Care Power of Attorney (Living Will)
- List of Allergic Reactions
- Organ Donor Card
- Social Security Card

In addition, save Business Cards from:

Doctors, Specialists, and Pharmacist.
Home Health Care provider.

Also Insurance Cards, noting 'first' or second insurance.

Either make copies and tape onto blank pages, or use a zippered pocket pouch, or file folder for easy storing.

Personal Information

Personal Information

Telephone Numbers and Addresses

Telephone Numbers and Addresses

As Mom grew weaker, she became easily confused and frustrated.

We called or visited her almost hourly. At certain times Mom would have an extreme amount of pain or discomfort. In her attempts to call us, and/or the doctor for advise or help, she often panicked trying to locate necessary phone numbers. This anxiety caused Mom's disposition to worsen.

For her convenience, we provided a page with all the phone numbers she used and needed. This included her own name, address and phone number because at any given moment she might be unable to think clearly when needing to make an emergency call.

Mom said this gave her a sense of ease, that enabled her to remain calm as she got in touch with whomever she needed to.

For emergency assistance, if needed.

Patient Name: _____
Address: _____
_____
Phone: _____

Emergency Contacts: **Relationship:** **Phone:**
   Name: _____ _____ _____
   Name: _____ _____ _____
   Name: _____ _____ _____
   Name: _____ _____ _____
   Name: _____ _____ _____

Doctor/Clinic: _____
   Address: _____
_____
   Phone: _____ Pager: _____
   Office contacts: _____

Hospital:
   Address: _____
_____
   Phone: _____

Insurance Information:
   Company: _____
   Phone: _____
   Group No.: _____

Insurance Information:
   Company: _____
   Phone: _____
   Group No.: _____

Specialist: _____
   Address: _____
   _____
   Phone: _____ Pager: _____
   Office contacts: _____

Specialist: _____
   Address: _____
   _____
   Phone: _____ Pager: _____
   Office contacts: _____

Pharmacy: _____
   Address: _____
   Phone: _____
   Pharmacist: _____
   Hours: _____

In-Home Care: _____
   Phone: _____ Pager: _____
   Office contacts: _____

In-Home Care: _____
   Phone: _____ Pager: _____
   Office contacts: _____

Other:
   Name: _____
   Address: _____
   Phone: _____ Pager: _____
   Office contacts: _____

   Name: _____
   Address: _____
   Phone: _____ Pager: _____
   Office contacts: _____

   Name: _____
   Address: _____
   Phone: _____ Pager: _____
   Office contacts: _____

Important Information

Appointment Calendar

Section 1

Appointment Calendar

Keeping track of all appointments on a calendar helped Mom to organize a schedule of when and where she needed to be.

Some months had little activity, while other months were filled with various types of appointments.

This fill-in type of calendar helped us manage our time and prevented doubling up on appointments. Mom easily kept track of who would be available to accompany her.

Some items written on Mom's calendar:

- Blood tests
- Chemotherapy
- Doctor appointments
- Duration of hospital stays
- Group Therapy
- In-Home Health Care
- Infusion Center
- Pain Management Group
- Prescriptions ready at pharmacy
- Scheduled surgery dates
- Specialists appointments
- X-rays

Appointment Calendar

Month/Yr: Jan 1995

Sun	Mon	Tue	Wed	Thu	Fri	Sat
1	2 Lab tests	3	4	5 home health nurse	6	7
8	9	10	11 Doctor 8:30 am	12 home health nurse	13	14
15 went to hospital emergency - for pain 2 p.m.	16	17	18	19 home health nurse	20	21
22	23	24 CAT Scan	25	26 home health nurse	27	28
29	30	31				

SAMPLE PAGE

Appointment Calendar

Month/Yr:

Sun	Mon	Tue	Wed	Thu	Fri	Sat

Appointment Calendar

Month/Yr:

Sun	Mon	Tue	Wed	Thu	Fri	Sat

Appointment Calendar

Month/Yr:

Sun	Mon	Tue	Wed	Thu	Fri	Sat

Appointment Calendar

Month/Yr:

Sun	Mon	Tue	Wed	Thu	Fri	Sat

Appointment Calendar

Month/Yr:

Sun	Mon	Tue	Wed	Thu	Fri	Sat

Appointment Calendar

Month/Yr:

Sun	Mon	Tue	Wed	Thu	Fri	Sat

Appointment Calendar

Month/Yr:

Sun	Mon	Tue	Wed	Thu	Fri	Sat

Appointment Calendar

Month/Yr:

Sun	Mon	Tue	Wed	Thu	Fri	Sat

Appointment Calendar

Month/Yr:

Sun	Mon	Tue	Wed	Thu	Fri	Sat

Appointment Calendar

Month/Yr:

Sun	Mon	Tue	Wed	Thu	Fri	Sat

Appointment Calendar

Month/Yr:

Sun	Mon	Tue	Wed	Thu	Fri	Sat

Appointment Calendar

Month/Yr:

Sun	Mon	Tue	Wed	Thu	Fri	Sat

Daily Health Chart

Section 2

Daily Health Chart

Throughout Mom's illness, she recorded information... important to both her and to the Doctor(s).

Recording her condition on a daily basis made the information readily available for reference.

In addition to the descriptions on the sample page, Mom recorded her status regarding:

- Appetite
- Blood pressure and pulse
- Bowel movement (amount and type)
- Breathing
- Fatigue
- Mood
- Nausea
- Pain
- Sleep
- Stomach ache
- Temperature
- Urine (amount and type)

> You may want to ask your Doctor what items would be helpful to record.

Daily Health Chart

Month/Year: June 1995

Day	Sun	Mon	Tue	Wed	Thu	Fri	Sat
Date	18	19	20	21	22	23	24

Description	Details						
Temperature	100.9	—	—	—	97.5	97.1	—
weight	123	—	—	123	—	—	—
bowel movement	Small, normal 11:45 a.m.	—	Runny 5:00 pm	—	—	Large amount *Bloody* 6:00 p.m.	—
urine	normal	→	→	→	→	→	→
daily activities	church am	Lunch out	rested	visitors in	grocery store	rested	rested
just don't feel good	—	—	—	—	—	bad day	bad day

SAMPLE PAGE

Daily Health Chart   Month/Year: _____

Day Date	Sun	Mon	Tue	Wed	Thu	Fri	Sat

Description	Details						

Daily Health Chart

Month/Year: _____

Day	Sun	Mon	Tue	Wed	Thu	Fri	Sat
Date							

Description	Details						

Daily Health Chart   Month/Year: _____

Day	Sun	Mon	Tue	Wed	Thu	Fri	Sat
Date							

Description	Details						

Daily Health Chart   Month/Year: _____

Day	Sun	Mon	Tue	Wed	Thu	Fri	Sat
Date							

Description	Details						

Daily Health Chart   Month/Year: _____

Day	Sun	Mon	Tue	Wed	Thu	Fri	Sat
Date							

Description	Details						

Daily Health Chart   Month/Year: _____

Day	Sun	Mon	Tue	Wed	Thu	Fri	Sat
Date							

Description	Details						

Daily Health Chart

Month/Year: _____

Day	Sun	Mon	Tue	Wed	Thu	Fri	Sat
Date							

Description	Details						

Daily Health Chart

Month/Year: _____

Day	Sun	Mon	Tue	Wed	Thu	Fri	Sat
Date							

Description	Details						

Daily Health Chart   Month/Year: _____

Day	Sun	Mon	Tue	Wed	Thu	Fri	Sat
Date							

Description	Details						

Daily Health Chart   Month/Year: _____

Day	Sun	Mon	Tue	Wed	Thu	Fri	Sat
Date							

Description	Details						

Daily Health Chart   Month/Year: _____

Day	Sun	Mon	Tue	Wed	Thu	Fri	Sat
Date							

Description	Details						

Daily Health Chart   Month/Year: _____

Day Date	Sun	Mon	Tue	Wed	Thu	Fri	Sat

Description	Details						

Daily Health Chart   Month/Year: _____

Day	Sun	Mon	Tue	Wed	Thu	Fri	Sat
Date							

Description	Details						

Daily Health Chart   Month/Year: _____

Day	Sun	Mon	Tue	Wed	Thu	Fri	Sat
Date							

Description	Details						

Daily Health Chart   Month/Year: _____

Day	Sun	Mon	Tue	Wed	Thu	Fri	Sat
Date							

Description	Details						

Daily Health Chart

Month/Year: _____

Day	Sun	Mon	Tue	Wed	Thu	Fri	Sat
Date							

Description	Details						

Daily Health Chart   Month/Year: _____

Day	Sun	Mon	Tue	Wed	Thu	Fri	Sat
Date							

Description	Details						

Daily Health Chart

Month/Year: _____

Day	Sun	Mon	Tue	Wed	Thu	Fri	Sat
Date							

Description	Details						

Daily Health Chart

Month/Year: _____

Day	Sun	Mon	Tue	Wed	Thu	Fri	Sat
Date							

Description	Details						

Daily Health Chart

Month/Year: _____

Day	Sun	Mon	Tue	Wed	Thu	Fri	Sat
Date							

Description	Details						

Daily Health Chart   Month/Year: _____

Day	Sun	Mon	Tue	Wed	Thu	Fri	Sat
Date							

Description	Details						

Daily Health Chart   Month/Year: _____

Day	Sun	Mon	Tue	Wed	Thu	Fri	Sat
Date							

Description	Details						

Daily Health Chart   Month/Year: _____

Day	Sun	Mon	Tue	Wed	Thu	Fri	Sat
Date							

Description	Details						

Daily Health Chart

Month/Year: _____

Day	Sun	Mon	Tue	Wed	Thu	Fri	Sat
Date							

Description	Details						

Daily Health Chart   Month/Year: _____

Day	Sun	Mon	Tue	Wed	Thu	Fri	Sat
Date							

Description	Details						

Daily Health Chart

Month/Year: _____

Day	Sun	Mon	Tue	Wed	Thu	Fri	Sat
Date							

Description	Details						

Daily Health Chart

Month/Year: _____

Day	Sun	Mon	Tue	Wed	Thu	Fri	Sat
Date							

Description	Details						

Daily Health Chart   Month/Year: _____

Day	Sun	Mon	Tue	Wed	Thu	Fri	Sat
Date							

Description	Details						

Daily Health Chart   Month/Year: _____

Day	Sun	Mon	Tue	Wed	Thu	Fri	Sat
Date							

Description	Details						

Daily Health Chart   Month/Year: _____

Day	Sun	Mon	Tue	Wed	Thu	Fri	Sat
Date							

Description	Details						

Daily Health Chart

Month/Year: _____

Day	Sun	Mon	Tue	Wed	Thu	Fri	Sat
Date							

Description	Details						

Daily Health Chart

Month/Year: _____

Day	Sun	Mon	Tue	Wed	Thu	Fri	Sat
Date							

Description	Details						

Daily Health Chart   Month/Year: _____

Day	Sun	Mon	Tue	Wed	Thu	Fri	Sat
Date							

Description	Details						

Daily Health Chart

Month/Year: _____

Day	Sun	Mon	Tue	Wed	Thu	Fri	Sat
Date							

Description	Details						

Daily Health Chart   Month/Year: _____

Day	Sun	Mon	Tue	Wed	Thu	Fri	Sat
Date							

Description	Details						

Daily Health Chart   Month/Year: _____

Day	Sun	Mon	Tue	Wed	Thu	Fri	Sat
Date							

Description	Details						

Daily Health Chart   Month/Year: _____

Day	Sun	Mon	Tue	Wed	Thu	Fri	Sat
Date							

Description	Details						

Daily Health Chart   Month/Year: _____

Day	Sun	Mon	Tue	Wed	Thu	Fri	Sat
Date							

Description	Details						

Daily Health Chart

Month/Year: _____

Day	Sun	Mon	Tue	Wed	Thu	Fri	Sat
Date							

Description	Details						

Daily Health Chart

Month/Year: _____

Day	Sun	Mon	Tue	Wed	Thu	Fri	Sat
Date							

Description	Details						

Daily Health Chart   Month/Year: _____

Day	Sun	Mon	Tue	Wed	Thu	Fri	Sat
Date							

Description	Details						

Daily Health Chart   Month/Year: _____

Day	Sun	Mon	Tue	Wed	Thu	Fri	Sat
Date							

Description	Details						

Daily Health Chart   Month/Year: _____

Day	Sun	Mon	Tue	Wed	Thu	Fri	Sat
Date							

Description	Details						

Daily Health Chart

Month/Year: _____

Day	Sun	Mon	Tue	Wed	Thu	Fri	Sat
Date							

Description	Details						

Daily Health Chart

Month/Year: _____

Day	Sun	Mon	Tue	Wed	Thu	Fri	Sat
Date							

Description	Details						

Daily Health Chart   Month/Year: _____

Day	Sun	Mon	Tue	Wed	Thu	Fri	Sat
Date							

Description	Details						

Daily Health Chart   Month/Year: _____

Day	Sun	Mon	Tue	Wed	Thu	Fri	Sat
Date							

Description	Details						

Daily Health Chart Month/Year: _____

Day	Sun	Mon	Tue	Wed	Thu	Fri	Sat
Date							

Description	Details						

Daily Health Chart   Month/Year: _____

Day	Sun	Mon	Tue	Wed	Thu	Fri	Sat
Date							

Description	Details						

Daily Health Chart   Month/Year: _____

Day	Sun	Mon	Tue	Wed	Thu	Fri	Sat
Date							

Description	Details						

Daily Health Chart   Month/Year: _____

Day	Sun	Mon	Tue	Wed	Thu	Fri	Sat
Date							

Description	Details						

Daily Health Chart   Month/Year: _____

Day	Sun	Mon	Tue	Wed	Thu	Fri	Sat
Date							

Description	Details						

Daily Medication Log

Section 3

Daily Medication Log

<u>Writing down the times Mom took medication became the most important section in the book.</u>

There were times Mom thought she had taken her medicine, but before anyone realized she had not, Mom went off schedule and often experienced a lot of unnecessary pain.

There were other times when Mom did take her medication and a short while later became confused, not being able to remember if she actually had taken the proper prescribed dosage. Mom would then take another tablet, not realizing she was doubling up on her medication.

To keep Mom from endangering herself, this log was created for her safety.

This section became our source of information as to what, when, and why Mom took medication. We were able to evaluate, at home, whether or not the medication helped and if she needed an increased dosage or strength.

> You may want to ask your Doctor what items would be helpful for you to record.

Daily Medication Log

Month/Year: _Sept 1995_

Day	Sun	Mon	Tue	Wed	Thu	Fri	Sat
Date	24	25	26	27	28	29	30

Medication	Details						
Name of medication, strength, dosage, usage, prescribed time(s)							
XYZ Tablet, 500 mg, 3 times a day for pain	—	—	—	8:30 a.m. NOON 5 p.m.	8:30 a.m. NOON 5 p.m.	8:30 a.m. NOON 5 p.m.	8:30 a.m. NOON 5 p.m.
IN HOSPITAL — chemotherapy medication used and dosage.	→						

105

SAMPLE PAGE

Daily Medication Log   Month/Year: _____

Day	Sun	Mon	Tue	Wed	Thu	Fri	Sat
Date							

Medication	Details					

Daily Medication Log   Month/Year: _____

Day	Sun	Mon	Tue	Wed	Thu	Fri	Sat
Date							

Medication	Details						

Daily Medication Log   Month/Year: _____

Day	Sun	Mon	Tue	Wed	Thu	Fri	Sat
Date							

Medication	Details						

Daily Medication Log   Month/Year: _____

Day	Sun	Mon	Tue	Wed	Thu	Fri	Sat
Date							

Medication	Details						

Daily Medication Log   Month/Year: _____

Day	Sun	Mon	Tue	Wed	Thu	Fri	Sat
Date							

Medication	Details						

Daily Medication Log   Month/Year: _____

Day	Sun	Mon	Tue	Wed	Thu	Fri	Sat
Date							

Medication	Details						

Daily Medication Log   Month/Year: _____

Day	Sun	Mon	Tue	Wed	Thu	Fri	Sat
Date							

Medication	Details					

Daily Medication Log   Month/Year: _____

Day	Sun	Mon	Tue	Wed	Thu	Fri	Sat
Date							

Medication	Details						

Daily Medication Log   Month/Year: _____

Day	Sun	Mon	Tue	Wed	Thu	Fri	Sat
Date							

Medication	Details						

Daily Medication Log   Month/Year: _____

Day	Sun	Mon	Tue	Wed	Thu	Fri	Sat
Date							

Medication	Details						

Daily Medication Log   Month/Year: _____

Day Date	Sun	Mon	Tue	Wed	Thu	Fri	Sat

Medication	Details						

Daily Medication Log   Month/Year: _____

Day	Sun	Mon	Tue	Wed	Thu	Fri	Sat
Date							

Medication	Details						

Daily Medication Log   Month/Year: _____

Day	Sun	Mon	Tue	Wed	Thu	Fri	Sat
Date							

Medication	Details						

Daily Medication Log   Month/Year: _____

Day	Sun	Mon	Tue	Wed	Thu	Fri	Sat
Date							

Medication	Details					

Daily Medication Log   Month/Year: _____

Day	Sun	Mon	Tue	Wed	Thu	Fri	Sat
Date							

Medication	Details						

Daily Medication Log   Month/Year: _____

Day	Sun	Mon	Tue	Wed	Thu	Fri	Sat
Date							

Medication	Details						

Daily Medication Log   Month/Year: _____

Day	Sun	Mon	Tue	Wed	Thu	Fri	Sat
Date							

Medication	Details						

Daily Medication Log   Month/Year: _____

Day	Sun	Mon	Tue	Wed	Thu	Fri	Sat
Date							

Medication	Details						

Daily Medication Log   Month/Year: _____

Day	Sun	Mon	Tue	Wed	Thu	Fri	Sat
Date							

Medication	Details						

Daily Medication Log   Month/Year: _____

Day	Sun	Mon	Tue	Wed	Thu	Fri	Sat
Date							

Medication	Details					

Daily Medication Log   Month/Year: _____

Day	Sun	Mon	Tue	Wed	Thu	Fri	Sat
Date							

Medication	Details						

Daily Medication Log   Month/Year: _____

Day	Sun	Mon	Tue	Wed	Thu	Fri	Sat
Date							

Medication	Details						

Daily Medication Log   Month/Year: _____

Day	Sun	Mon	Tue	Wed	Thu	Fri	Sat
Date							

Medication	Details						

Daily Medication Log   Month/Year: _____

Day	Sun	Mon	Tue	Wed	Thu	Fri	Sat
Date							

Medication	Details						

Daily Medication Log   Month/Year: _____

Day	Sun	Mon	Tue	Wed	Thu	Fri	Sat
Date							

Medication	Details						

Daily Medication Log   Month/Year: _____

Day	Sun	Mon	Tue	Wed	Thu	Fri	Sat
Date							

Medication	Details						

Daily Medication Log   Month/Year: _____

Day	Sun	Mon	Tue	Wed	Thu	Fri	Sat
Date							

Medication	Details						

Daily Medication Log   Month/Year: _____

Day	Sun	Mon	Tue	Wed	Thu	Fri	Sat
Date							

Medication	Details						

Daily Medication Log

Month/Year: _____

Day	Sun	Mon	Tue	Wed	Thu	Fri	Sat
Date							

Medication	Details						

Daily Medication Log   Month/Year: _____

Day	Sun	Mon	Tue	Wed	Thu	Fri	Sat
Date							

Medication	Details						

Daily Medication Log

Month/Year: _____

Day	Sun	Mon	Tue	Wed	Thu	Fri	Sat
Date							

Medication	Details						

Daily Medication Log   Month/Year: _____

Day	Sun	Mon	Tue	Wed	Thu	Fri	Sat
Date							

Medication	Details						

Daily Medication Log   Month/Year: _____

Day	Sun	Mon	Tue	Wed	Thu	Fri	Sat
Date							

Medication	Details						

Daily Medication Log   Month/Year: _____

Day	Sun	Mon	Tue	Wed	Thu	Fri	Sat
Date							

Medication	Details						

Daily Medication Log   Month/Year: _____

Day	Sun	Mon	Tue	Wed	Thu	Fri	Sat
Date							

Medication	Details						

Daily Medication Log Month/Year: _____

Day	Sun	Mon	Tue	Wed	Thu	Fri	Sat
Date							

Medication	Details						

Daily Medication Log   Month/Year: _____

Day	Sun	Mon	Tue	Wed	Thu	Fri	Sat
Date							

Medication	Details						

Daily Medication Log   Month/Year: _____

Day	Sun	Mon	Tue	Wed	Thu	Fri	Sat
Date							

Medication	Details						

Daily Medication Log   Month/Year: _____

Day	Sun	Mon	Tue	Wed	Thu	Fri	Sat
Date							

Medication	Details						

Daily Medication Log   Month/Year: _____

Day Date	Sun	Mon	Tue	Wed	Thu	Fri	Sat

Medication	Details						

Daily Medication Log   Month/Year: _____

Day	Sun	Mon	Tue	Wed	Thu	Fri	Sat
Date							

Medication	Details						

Daily Medication Log   Month/Year: _____

Day	Sun	Mon	Tue	Wed	Thu	Fri	Sat
Date							

Medication	Details						

Daily Medication Log   Month/Year: _____

Day	Sun	Mon	Tue	Wed	Thu	Fri	Sat
Date							

Medication	Details						

Daily Medication Log Month/Year: _____

Day	Sun	Mon	Tue	Wed	Thu	Fri	Sat
Date							

Medication	Details						

Daily Medication Log   Month/Year: _____

Day	Sun	Mon	Tue	Wed	Thu	Fri	Sat
Date							

Medication	Details						

Daily Medication Log   Month/Year: _____

Day	Sun	Mon	Tue	Wed	Thu	Fri	Sat
Date							

Medication	Details						

Daily Medication Log   Month/Year: _____

Day Date	Sun	Mon	Tue	Wed	Thu	Fri	Sat

Medication	Details						

Daily Medication Log   Month/Year: _____

Day Date	Sun	Mon	Tue	Wed	Thu	Fri	Sat

Medication	Details						

Daily Medication Log   Month/Year: _____

Day	Sun	Mon	Tue	Wed	Thu	Fri	Sat
Date							

Medication	Details						

Daily Medication Log   Month/Year: _____

Day	Sun	Mon	Tue	Wed	Thu	Fri	Sat
Date							

Medication	Details						

Daily Medication Log   Month/Year: _____

Day	Sun	Mon	Tue	Wed	Thu	Fri	Sat
Date							

Medication	Details						

Daily Medication Log   Month/Year: _____

Day	Sun	Mon	Tue	Wed	Thu	Fri	Sat
Date							

Medication	Details						

Medicine

Section 4

Medicine

This section is designed to record comments regarding each prescribed medicine.

During the course of Mom's illness, she took numerous medications. Whether prescribed for pain, anxiety, or whatever the case, she kept a close account of the details, which proved beneficial.

Mom was able to tolerate some medications, but not others.

For instance, Mother could not handle one drug because it made her nauseated. Keeping track worked out well for us. The doctor prescribed a different medicine that ultimately worked better for her.

A year later, she was in a situation that called for that same medication again. Since we had kept track, we were able to look back through this section to quickly realize she wouldn't be able to tolerate that particular medication. It made it easy for the doctor to prescribe an alternative medication.

Drugs used in Chemotherapy or treatments, and their side effects, if any, can be noted in this section.

This page will help you record detailed information prescribed medications.

Medication Name: _____
Dose: _____
Date Began: _____
Reason: _____
Date Stopped: _____
Reason/Reaction: _____

Medication Name: _____
Dose: _____
Date Began: _____
Reason: _____
Date Stopped: _____
Reason/Reaction: _____

Medication Name: _____
Dose: _____
Date Began: _____
Reason: _____
Date Stopped: _____
Reason/Reaction: _____

Medication Name: _____
Dose: _____
Date Began: _____
Reason: _____
Date Stopped: _____
Reason/Reaction: _____

This page will help you record detailed information prescribed medications.

Medication Name: _____
Dose: _____
Date Began: _____
Reason: _____
Date Stopped: _____
Reason/Reaction: _____

Medication Name: _____
Dose: _____
Date Began: _____
Reason: _____
Date Stopped: _____
Reason/Reaction: _____

Medication Name: _____
Dose: _____
Date Began: _____
Reason: _____
Date Stopped: _____
Reason/Reaction: _____

Medication Name: _____
Dose: _____
Date Began: _____
Reason: _____
Date Stopped: _____
Reason/Reaction: _____

This page will help you record detailed information prescribed medications.

Medication Name: _____
Dose: _____
Date Began: _____
Reason: _____
Date Stopped: _____
Reason/Reaction: _____

Medication Name: _____
Dose: _____
Date Began: _____
Reason: _____
Date Stopped: _____
Reason/Reaction: _____

Medication Name: _____
Dose: _____
Date Began: _____
Reason: _____
Date Stopped: _____
Reason/Reaction: _____

Medication Name: _____
Dose: _____
Date Began: _____
Reason: _____
Date Stopped: _____
Reason/Reaction: _____

This page will help you record detailed information prescribed medications.

Medication Name: _____
Dose: _____
Date Began: _____
Reason: _____
Date Stopped: _____
Reason/Reaction: _____
_____

Medication Name: _____
Dose: _____
Date Began: _____
Reason: _____
Date Stopped: _____
Reason/Reaction: _____
_____

Medication Name: _____
Dose: _____
Date Began: _____
Reason: _____
Date Stopped: _____
Reason/Reaction: _____
_____

Medication Name: _____
Dose: _____
Date Began: _____
Reason: _____
Date Stopped: _____
Reason/Reaction: _____
_____

This page will help you record detailed information prescribed medications.

Medication Name: _____
Dose: _____
Date Began: _____
Reason: _____
Date Stopped: _____
Reason/Reaction: _____

Medication Name: _____
Dose: _____
Date Began: _____
Reason: _____
Date Stopped: _____
Reason/Reaction: _____

Medication Name: _____
Dose: _____
Date Began: _____
Reason: _____
Date Stopped: _____
Reason/Reaction: _____

Medication Name: _____
Dose: _____
Date Began: _____
Reason: _____
Date Stopped: _____
Reason/Reaction: _____

This page will help you record detailed information prescribed medications.

Medication Name: _____
Dose: _____
Date Began: _____
Reason: _____
Date Stopped: _____
Reason/Reaction: _____

Medication Name: _____
Dose: _____
Date Began: _____
Reason: _____
Date Stopped: _____
Reason/Reaction: _____

Medication Name: _____
Dose: _____
Date Began: _____
Reason: _____
Date Stopped: _____
Reason/Reaction: _____

Medication Name: _____
Dose: _____
Date Began: _____
Reason: _____
Date Stopped: _____
Reason/Reaction: _____

This page will help you record detailed information prescribed medications.

Medication Name: _____
Dose: _____
Date Began: _____
Reason: _____
Date Stopped: _____
Reason/Reaction: _____

Medication Name: _____
Dose: _____
Date Began: _____
Reason: _____
Date Stopped: _____
Reason/Reaction: _____

Medication Name: _____
Dose: _____
Date Began: _____
Reason: _____
Date Stopped: _____
Reason/Reaction: _____

Medication Name: _____
Dose: _____
Date Began: _____
Reason: _____
Date Stopped: _____
Reason/Reaction: _____

This page will help you record detailed information prescribed medications.

Medication Name: _____
Dose: _____
Date Began: _____
Reason: _____
Date Stopped: _____
Reason/Reaction: _____
_____

Medication Name: _____
Dose: _____
Date Began: _____
Reason: _____
Date Stopped: _____
Reason/Reaction: _____
_____

Medication Name: _____
Dose: _____
Date Began: _____
Reason: _____
Date Stopped: _____
Reason/Reaction: _____
_____

Medication Name: _____
Dose: _____
Date Began: _____
Reason: _____
Date Stopped: _____
Reason/Reaction: _____
_____

This page will help you record detailed information prescribed medications.

Medication Name: _____
Dose: _____
Date Began: _____
Reason: _____
Date Stopped: _____
Reason/Reaction: _____

Medication Name: _____
Dose: _____
Date Began: _____
Reason: _____
Date Stopped: _____
Reason/Reaction: _____

Medication Name: _____
Dose: _____
Date Began: _____
Reason: _____
Date Stopped: _____
Reason/Reaction: _____

Medication Name: _____
Dose: _____
Date Began: _____
Reason: _____
Date Stopped: _____
Reason/Reaction: _____

This page will help you record detailed information prescribed medications.

Medication Name: _____
Dose: _____
Date Began: _____
Reason: _____
Date Stopped: _____
Reason/Reaction: _____
_____

Medication Name: _____
Dose: _____
Date Began: _____
Reason: _____
Date Stopped: _____
Reason/Reaction: _____
_____

Medication Name: _____
Dose: _____
Date Began: _____
Reason: _____
Date Stopped: _____
Reason/Reaction: _____
_____

Medication Name: _____
Dose: _____
Date Began: _____
Reason: _____
Date Stopped: _____
Reason/Reaction: _____
_____

Questions for the Doctor

Section 5

Questions

This section is useful for recording questions in preparing for appointments, phone communication, or for talks with the pharmacist. When test results, diagnoses, etc., are discussed, you will have reminders for necessary, pertinent questions.

The space on the following pages is provided to record your questions and later, their answers. Write them down as they come to mind.

Facts and information can sometimes become overwhelming and difficult to take in all at once. It can be confusing. Don't be too shy to ask how to spell medical words, terms, and procedures, or to have something reexplained or clarified.

Some questions we asked:

What type of cancer does Mom have?

What is your long-term plan......short-term plan?

What type of treatments are available?

Will a heating pad help?

What are the side affects to.....?

What caused.....?

Questions for Professional Persons/Caregivers

Date:
To:

Question:

Notes:

Date:
To:

Question:

Notes:

Date:
To:

Question:

Notes:

Questions for Professional Persons/Caregivers

Date: _____
To: _____

Question: _____
_____
_____

Notes: _____
_____
_____
_____

Date: _____
To: _____

Question: _____
_____
_____

Notes: _____
_____
_____
_____

Date: _____
To: _____

Question: _____
_____
_____

Notes: _____
_____
_____
_____

Questions for Professional Persons/Caregivers

Date:
To: _____

Question: _____
_____
_____
_____

Notes: _____
_____
_____
_____

Date:
To: _____

Question: _____
_____
_____
_____

Notes: _____
_____
_____
_____

Date:
To: _____

Question: _____
_____
_____
_____

Notes: _____
_____
_____
_____

Questions for Professional Persons/Caregivers

Date:
To:

Question:

Notes:

Date:
To:

Question:

Notes:

Date:
To:

Question:

Notes:

Questions for Professional Persons/Caregivers

Date: _____
To: _____

Question: _____
_____
_____

Notes: _____
_____
_____
_____

Date: _____
To: _____

Question: _____
_____
_____

Notes: _____
_____
_____
_____

Date: _____
To: _____

Question: _____
_____
_____

Notes: _____
_____
_____
_____

Questions for Professional Persons/Caregivers

Date: _____
To: _____

Question: _____
_____
_____

Notes: _____
_____
_____
_____

Date: _____
To: _____

Question: _____
_____
_____

Notes: _____
_____
_____
_____

Date: _____
To: _____

Question: _____
_____
_____

Notes: _____
_____
_____
_____

Questions for Professional Persons/Caregivers

Date: _____
To: _____

Question: _____
_____
_____

Notes: _____
_____
_____
_____

Date: _____
To: _____

Question: _____
_____
_____

Notes: _____
_____
_____
_____

Date: _____
To: _____

Question: _____
_____
_____

Notes: _____
_____
_____
_____

Questions for Professional Persons/Caregivers

Date: _____
To: _____

Question: _____
_____
_____

Notes: _____
_____
_____
_____

Date: _____
To: _____

Question: _____
_____
_____

Notes: _____
_____
_____
_____

Date: _____
To: _____

Question: _____
_____
_____

Notes: _____
_____
_____
_____

Questions for Professional Persons/Caregivers

Date: _____
To: _____

Question: _____
_____
_____

Notes: _____
_____
_____
_____

Date: _____
To: _____

Question: _____
_____
_____

Notes: _____
_____
_____
_____

Date: _____
To: _____

Question: _____
_____
_____

Notes: _____
_____
_____

Questions for Professional Persons/Caregivers

Date:
To:

Question:

Notes:

Date:
To:

Question:

Notes:

Date:
To:

Question:

Notes:

Tests and Results

Section 6

Tests, Lab Results and Assessments

Mom's illness perpetuated various types of tests, such as Blood Counts, C.A.T. Scans, and X-rays.

Recording laboratory results help in the comprehension of issues relating to the illness, and also makes helpful information conveniently available for the doctor(s), on-call doctor, emergency care staff, and all health care team members.

The compiled data is useful in subsequent testing visits, and makes the technicians aware that you are familiar with the procedure.

Test items to document:

- Date
- Type
- Reason
- Requesting Doctor or Specialist
- Location, building, department, or floor
- Results

Tests and Results

Date:
Type:
Reason:
Requested by:
Location:
Result/Evaluation:

Date:
Type:
Reason:
Requested by:
Location:
Result/Evaluation:

Date:
Type:
Reason:
Requested by:
Location:
Result/Evaluation:

Date:
Type:
Reason:
Requested by:
Location:
Result/Evaluation:

Tests and Results

Date: _____
Type: _____
Reason: _____
Requested by: _____
Location: _____
Result/Evaluation: _____
_____

Date: _____
Type: _____
Reason: _____
Requested by: _____
Location: _____
Result/Evaluation: _____
_____

Date: _____
Type: _____
Reason: _____
Requested by: _____
Location: _____
Result/Evaluation: _____
_____

Date: _____
Type: _____
Reason: _____
Requested by: _____
Location: _____
Result/Evaluation: _____
_____

Tests and Results

Date:
Type:
Reason:
Requested by:
Location:
Result/Evaluation:

Date:
Type:
Reason:
Requested by:
Location:
Result/Evaluation:

Date:
Type:
Reason:
Requested by:
Location:
Result/Evaluation:

Date:
Type:
Reason:
Requested by:
Location:
Result/Evaluation:

Tests and Results

Date:
Type:
Reason:
Requested by:
Location:
Result/Evaluation:

Date:
Type:
Reason:
Requested by:
Location:
Result/Evaluation:

Date:
Type:
Reason:
Requested by:
Location:
Result/Evaluation:

Date:
Type:
Reason:
Requested by:
Location:
Result/Evaluation:

Tests and Results

Date:
Type:
Reason:
Requested by:
Location:
Result/Evaluation:

Date:
Type:
Reason:
Requested by:
Location:
Result/Evaluation:

Date:
Type:
Reason:
Requested by:
Location:
Result/Evaluation:

Date:
Type:
Reason:
Requested by:
Location:
Result/Evaluation:

Tests and Results

Date:
Type:
Reason:
Requested by:
Location:
Result/Evaluation:

Date:
Type:
Reason:
Requested by:
Location:
Result/Evaluation:

Date:
Type:
Reason:
Requested by:
Location:
Result/Evaluation:

Date:
Type:
Reason:
Requested by:
Location:
Result/Evaluation:

Tests and Results

Date:
Type:
Reason:
Requested by:
Location:
Result/Evaluation:

Date:
Type:
Reason:
Requested by:
Location:
Result/Evaluation:

Date:
Type:
Reason:
Requested by:
Location:
Result/Evaluation:

Date:
Type:
Reason:
Requested by:
Location:
Result/Evaluation:

Tests and Results

Date:
Type:
Reason:
Requested by:
Location:
Result/Evaluation:

Date:
Type:
Reason:
Requested by:
Location:
Result/Evaluation:

Date:
Type:
Reason:
Requested by:
Location:
Result/Evaluation:

Date:
Type:
Reason:
Requested by:
Location:
Result/Evaluation:

Tests and Results

Date:
Type:
Reason:
Requested by:
Location:
Result/Evaluation:

_____

Date:
Type:
Reason:
Requested by:
Location:
Result/Evaluation:

_____

Date:
Type:
Reason:
Requested by:
Location:
Result/Evaluation:

_____

Date:
Type:
Reason:
Requested by:
Location:
Result/Evaluation:

Tests and Results

Date:
Type:
Reason:
Requested by:
Location:
Result/Evaluation:

Date:
Type:
Reason:
Requested by:
Location:
Result/Evaluation:

Date:
Type:
Reason:
Requested by:
Location:
Result/Evaluation:

Date:
Type:
Reason:
Requested by:
Location:
Result/Evaluation:

Surgery/Hospital Stay

Section 7

Surgery/Hospital Stay

Over a two year period, Mom had two major surgeries followed by radiation, implants and chemotherapy treatments.

We used the recorded data for various reasons to refer back to the dates of her hospitalization: type of treatment/surgery performed, discussions with doctors, and instructions on helping Mom recover at home.

The details of hospital pre-admission were also completely recorded ahead of the actual surgery day to ease Mom's tension, making the transition go smoother for her.

> You may also want to record Chemotherapy or treatment drug and dose administered in this section.

Dates and information regarding Hospitalization.

Date: _____
Reason: _____
Hospital: _____
Doctor(s): _____

Notes:

_____
_____
_____
_____
_____

Date: _____
Reason: _____
Hospital: _____
Doctor(s): _____

Notes:

_____
_____
_____
_____
_____

Date: _____
Reason: _____
Hospital: _____
Doctor(s): _____

Notes:

_____
_____
_____
_____
_____

Dates and information regarding Hospitalization.

Date: _____
Reason: _____
Hospital: _____
Doctor(s): _____

Notes:
_____
_____
_____
_____
_____

Date: _____
Reason: _____
Hospital: _____
Doctor(s): _____

Notes:
_____
_____
_____
_____
_____

Date: _____
Reason: _____
Hospital: _____
Doctor(s): _____

Notes:
_____
_____
_____
_____
_____

Dates and information regarding Hospitalization.

Date: _____
Reason: _____
Hospital: _____
Doctor(s): _____

Notes:

_____
_____
_____
_____

Date: _____
Reason: _____
Hospital: _____
Doctor(s): _____

Notes:

_____
_____
_____
_____

Date: _____
Reason: _____
Hospital: _____
Doctor(s): _____

Notes:

_____
_____
_____
_____

Dates and information regarding Hospitalization.

Date: _____
Reason: _____
Hospital: _____
Doctor(s): _____

Notes:
_____
_____
_____
_____
_____

Date: _____
Reason: _____
Hospital: _____
Doctor(s): _____

Notes:
_____
_____
_____
_____
_____

Date: _____
Reason: _____
Hospital: _____
Doctor(s): _____

Notes:
_____
_____
_____
_____
_____

Dates and information regarding Hospitalization.

Date: _____
Reason: _____
Hospital: _____
Doctor(s): _____

Notes:

_____
_____
_____
_____
_____

Date: _____
Reason: _____
Hospital: _____
Doctor(s): _____

Notes:

_____
_____
_____
_____
_____

Date: _____
Reason: _____
Hospital: _____
Doctor(s): _____

Notes:

_____
_____
_____
_____
_____

Dates and information regarding Hospitalization.

Date: _____
Reason: _____
Hospital: _____
Doctor(s): _____

Notes:

_____
_____
_____
_____
_____

Date: _____
Reason: _____
Hospital: _____
Doctor(s): _____

Notes:

_____
_____
_____
_____
_____

Date: _____
Reason: _____
Hospital: _____
Doctor(s): _____

Notes:

_____
_____
_____
_____
_____

Dates and information regarding Hospitalization.

Date: _____
Reason: _____
Hospital: _____
Doctor(s): _____

Notes:

_____
_____
_____
_____
_____

Date: _____
Reason: _____
Hospital: _____
Doctor(s): _____

Notes:

_____
_____
_____
_____
_____

Date: _____
Reason: _____
Hospital: _____
Doctor(s): _____

Notes:

_____
_____
_____
_____
_____

Dates and information regarding Hospitalization.

Date: _____

Reason: _____

Hospital: _____

Doctor(s): _____

Notes:

_____

_____

_____

_____

_____

Date: _____

Reason: _____

Hospital: _____

Doctor(s): _____

Notes:

_____

_____

_____

_____

_____

Date: _____

Reason: _____

Hospital: _____

Doctor(s): _____

Notes:

_____

_____

_____

_____

_____

Dates and information regarding Hospitalization.

Date: _____
Reason: _____
Hospital: _____
Doctor(s): _____

Notes:
_____
_____
_____
_____
_____

Date: _____
Reason: _____
Hospital: _____
Doctor(s): _____

Notes:
_____
_____
_____
_____
_____

Date: _____
Reason: _____
Hospital: _____
Doctor(s): _____

Notes:
_____
_____
_____
_____
_____

Dates and information regarding Hospitalization.

Date: _____

Reason: _____

Hospital: _____

Doctor(s): _____

Notes:

_____

_____

_____

_____

_____

Date: _____

Reason: _____

Hospital: _____

Doctor(s): _____

Notes:

_____

_____

_____

_____

_____

Date: _____

Reason: _____

Hospital: _____

Doctor(s): _____

Notes:

_____

_____

_____

_____

_____

Referrals

Section 8

Referrals

The Doctors, nurses, and office staff referred Mom to different places and groups for assistance, according to her needs.

Keeping a list of those names and/or places helped Mom in locating them without having to leave home.

Here are some types of referrals Mom recorded:

- Association's, Foundation's, Societies
- Beauty Supply Stores
- Medical Supply Stores
- Support Groups/Individuals

Referrals

Name: _____
Address: _____
Phone: ( ) _____
Contact: _____

Notes: _____
_____
_____
_____

Name: _____
Address: _____
Phone: ( ) _____
Contact: _____

Notes: _____
_____
_____
_____

Name: _____
Address: _____
Phone: ( ) _____
Contact: _____

Notes: _____
_____
_____
_____

Referrals

Name: _____
Address: _____
Phone: ( ) _____
Contact: _____

Notes: _____
_____
_____
_____

Name: _____
Address: _____
Phone: ( ) _____
Contact: _____

Notes: _____
_____
_____
_____

Name: _____
Address: _____
Phone: ( ) _____
Contact: _____

Notes: _____
_____
_____
_____

Referrals

Name: _____
Address: _____
Phone: ( ) _____
Contact: _____

Notes: _____
_____
_____
_____

Name: _____
Address: _____
Phone: ( ) _____
Contact: _____

Notes: _____
_____
_____
_____

Name: _____
Address: _____
Phone: ( ) _____
Contact: _____

Notes: _____
_____
_____
_____

Referrals

Name: _____
Address: _____
Phone: ( ) _____
Contact: _____

Notes: _____
_____
_____
_____

Name: _____
Address: _____
Phone: ( ) _____
Contact: _____

Notes: _____
_____
_____
_____

Name: _____
Address: _____
Phone: ( ) _____
Contact: _____

Notes: _____
_____
_____
_____

Referrals

Name: _____
Address: _____
Phone: ( ) _____
Contact: _____

Notes: _____
_____
_____
_____

Name: _____
Address: _____
Phone: ( ) _____
Contact: _____

Notes: _____
_____
_____
_____

Name: _____
Address: _____
Phone: ( ) _____
Contact: _____

Notes: _____
_____
_____
_____

Referrals

Name: _____
Address: _____
Phone: ( ) _____
Contact: _____

Notes: _____
_____
_____
_____

Name: _____
Address: _____
Phone: ( ) _____
Contact: _____

Notes: _____
_____
_____
_____

Name: _____
Address: _____
Phone: ( ) _____
Contact: _____

Notes: _____
_____
_____
_____

Referrals

Name: _____
Address: _____
Phone: ( ) _____
Contact: _____

Notes: _____
_____
_____
_____

Name: _____
Address: _____
Phone: ( ) _____
Contact: _____

Notes: _____
_____
_____
_____

Name: _____
Address: _____
Phone: ( ) _____
Contact: _____

Notes: _____
_____
_____
_____

Referrals

Name: _____
Address: _____
Phone: ( ) _____
Contact: _____

Notes: _____
_____
_____
_____

Name: _____
Address: _____
Phone: ( ) _____
Contact: _____

Notes: _____
_____
_____
_____

Name: _____
Address: _____
Phone: ( ) _____
Contact: _____

Notes: _____
_____
_____
_____

Referrals

Name: _____
Address: _____
Phone: ( ) _____
Contact: _____

Notes: _____
_____
_____
_____

Name: _____
Address: _____
Phone: ( ) _____
Contact: _____

Notes: _____
_____
_____
_____

Name: _____
Address: _____
Phone: ( ) _____
Contact: _____

Notes: _____
_____
_____
_____

Referrals

Name: _____
Address: _____
Phone: ( ) _____
Contact: _____

Notes: _____
_____
_____
_____

Name: _____
Address: _____
Phone: ( ) _____
Contact: _____

Notes: _____
_____
_____
_____

Name: _____
Address: _____
Phone: ( ) _____
Contact: _____

Notes: _____
_____
_____
_____

Helpful Hints

Section 9

Helpful Hints

Ideas, Advice and Suggestions to use during an illness and/or recovery.

This section is a family favorite. We continually discovered new ways of helping Mom make adjustments in order to make simple tasks easier.

Every time we entered into a different phase of Mom's illness, we would develop new ways to approach tasks. Mom would sometimes suggest how to improve a situation.

We became quite creative in our shortcuts by using our imagination and being flexible.

This section is unique to each individual's needs and can be helpful to everyone involved, when coming together during the hard times.*

*Note: If you would like to submit some of your own Helpful Hints for possible additions to the next revised "HopeWorks Medical Diary" see Section 14, under Comments and Suggestions.

Here are some samples of what worked for Mom.

If at all possible, take someone with you to every appointment and/or hospital visit. Have them take notes. They can review the doctors instructions with you later, if you are confused.

Use support bars and a shower chair in the bath/shower.

For a decreased appetite place 6 or 7 small portions of food on the plate for variety, instead of the regular three helpings.

Use a cane for pulling things toward you, closing doors, drawers, etc.

If your hands are cold, wear gloves to take things out of the refrigerator, and also wear them for grip to take off lids, to open boxes, etc.

For daily convenience, keep bottled water in every room.

Ask your doctor about getting a Handicap Parking Pass during your illness. Call the DMV for the form.

When seated on a low couch, chair, toilet, etc., put one foot a step ahead of the other, then lean forward to help you to get up easier.

If you have trouble with nausea, swallowing, or keeping medication down, ask your doctor if elixirs or rectal suppositories are available.

When appropriate, call a Cancer Society or other society and find out how they might help you.

Keep the radio on and tuned in to a pleasant sounding station...helps attitude, and loneliness.

Try to get out of the house at least once a day; perhaps a friend can take you for a ride around the block.

Keep moist towelettes beside the bed and/or near lounge chair, to easily clean hands without getting up—in case it's difficult.

If it becomes difficult to swallow pills, cut them in half or, dissolve in a small amount of water. If swallowing is still too difficult, use an eyedropper.

If mouth is dry, use a spray bottle to spray small amounts of water into the mouth.

Helpful Hints

Helpful Hints

Helpful Hints

Helpful Hints

Helpful Hints

Helpful Hints

Helpful Hints

Helpful Hints

Helpful Hints

Helpful Hints

Personal Diary

Section 10

Personal Diary

After Mom found out she had cancer, she kept a diary.

Sometimes she would journal everyday and other times it might be once a week.

It depended upon how she felt physically and whether or not she needed to express her emotions.

Here are some examples:

August 19th

Not feeling good. Can't concentrate. Eyes are blurred.

September 7th

Felt pretty good when I got up. After breakfast...began to feel bad. Back and leg hurt. Used heating pads. Didn't take medicine on time. Began to feel better at noon. Felt better in the evening, but fully tired when I went to bed. Still taking both pain pills.

September 14th

Showered - weak. Only ate half a bowl of cereal. Vomited twice. Took medicine all through the night. Felt weak. Enjoy having the kids take turns staying all night.

September 29th

Kids took me to infusion center for blood transfusion.

October 21

Slept late. Pain still same, leg swollen.

Diary

Date _____

_____
_____
_____
_____
_____

Date _____

_____
_____
_____
_____
_____

Date _____

_____
_____
_____
_____
_____

Date _____

_____
_____
_____
_____
_____

Date _____

_____
_____
_____
_____
_____

Diary

Date _____

_____
_____
_____
_____
_____

Date _____

_____
_____
_____
_____
_____
_____

Date _____

_____
_____
_____
_____
_____
_____

Date _____

_____
_____
_____
_____

Date _____

_____
_____
_____
_____
_____

Diary

Date _____

Date _____

Date _____

Date _____

Date _____

Diary

Date _____

_____
_____
_____
_____
_____

Date _____

_____
_____
_____
_____
_____

Date _____

_____
_____
_____
_____
_____

Date _____

_____
_____
_____
_____
_____

Date _____

_____
_____
_____
_____
_____

Diary

Date _____

_____
_____
_____
_____
_____

Date _____

_____
_____
_____
_____
_____
_____

Date _____

_____
_____
_____
_____
_____
_____

Date _____

_____
_____
_____
_____
_____

Date _____

_____
_____
_____
_____
_____

Diary

Date _____

_____
_____
_____
_____
_____

Date _____

_____
_____
_____
_____
_____
_____

Date _____

_____
_____
_____
_____
_____
_____

Date _____

_____
_____
_____
_____
_____

Date _____

_____
_____
_____
_____
_____

Diary

Date _____

_____
_____
_____
_____
_____
_____

Date _____

_____
_____
_____
_____
_____
_____

Date _____

_____
_____
_____
_____
_____
_____

Date _____

_____
_____
_____
_____
_____

Date _____

_____
_____
_____
_____
_____
_____

Diary

Date _____

_____
_____
_____
_____
_____
_____

Date _____

_____
_____
_____
_____
_____
_____

Date _____

_____
_____
_____
_____
_____
_____

Date _____

_____
_____
_____
_____
_____

Date _____

_____
_____
_____
_____
_____

Diary

Date _____

Date _____

Date _____

Date _____

Date _____

Diary

Date _____

_____
_____
_____
_____
_____
_____

Date _____

_____
_____
_____
_____
_____
_____

Date _____

_____
_____
_____
_____
_____
_____

Date _____

_____
_____
_____
_____
_____
_____

Date _____

_____
_____
_____
_____
_____
_____

Diary

Date _____

_____
_____
_____
_____
_____

Date _____

_____
_____
_____
_____
_____
_____

Date _____

_____
_____
_____
_____
_____
_____

Date _____

_____
_____
_____
_____
_____

Date _____

_____
_____
_____
_____
_____

Diary

Date _____

_____
_____
_____
_____
_____
_____

Date _____

_____
_____
_____
_____
_____
_____

Date _____

_____
_____
_____
_____
_____
_____

Date _____

_____
_____
_____
_____
_____

Date _____

_____
_____
_____
_____
_____

Diary

Date _____

_____
_____
_____
_____
_____
_____

Date _____

_____
_____
_____
_____
_____
_____

Date _____

_____
_____
_____
_____
_____
_____

Date _____

_____
_____
_____
_____
_____

Date _____

_____
_____
_____
_____
_____

Diary

Date _____

_____
_____
_____
_____
_____
_____

Date _____

_____
_____
_____
_____
_____
_____

Date _____

_____
_____
_____
_____
_____
_____

Date _____

_____
_____
_____
_____
_____

Date _____

_____
_____
_____
_____
_____
_____

Diary

Date _____

_____
_____
_____
_____
_____

Date _____

_____
_____
_____
_____
_____

Date _____

_____
_____
_____
_____
_____

Date _____

_____
_____
_____
_____
_____

Date _____

_____
_____
_____
_____
_____

Diary

Date _____

_____
_____
_____
_____
_____

Date _____

_____
_____
_____
_____
_____

Date _____

_____
_____
_____
_____
_____

Date _____

_____
_____
_____
_____
_____

Date _____

_____
_____
_____
_____
_____

Diary

Date _____

_____
_____
_____
_____
_____

Date _____

_____
_____
_____
_____
_____

Date _____

_____
_____
_____
_____
_____

Date _____

_____
_____
_____
_____
_____

Date _____

_____
_____
_____
_____
_____

Diary

Date _____

_____
_____
_____
_____
_____

Date _____

_____
_____
_____
_____
_____

Date _____

_____
_____
_____
_____
_____

Date _____

_____
_____
_____
_____
_____

Date _____

_____
_____
_____
_____
_____

Diary

Date _____

_____
_____
_____
_____
_____
_____

Date _____

_____
_____
_____
_____
_____
_____

Date _____

_____
_____
_____
_____
_____
_____

Date _____

_____
_____
_____
_____
_____

Date _____

_____
_____
_____
_____
_____

Diary

Date _____

_____
_____
_____
_____
_____

Date _____

_____
_____
_____
_____
_____

Date _____

_____
_____
_____
_____
_____

Date _____

_____
_____
_____
_____
_____

Date _____

_____
_____
_____
_____
_____

Diary

Date _____

_____
_____
_____
_____
_____

Date _____

_____
_____
_____
_____
_____

Date _____

_____
_____
_____
_____
_____

Date _____

_____
_____
_____
_____
_____

Date _____

_____
_____
_____
_____
_____

Diary

Date _____

_____
_____
_____
_____
_____
_____

Date _____

_____
_____
_____
_____
_____
_____

Date _____

_____
_____
_____
_____
_____
_____

Date _____

_____
_____
_____
_____
_____
_____

Date _____

_____
_____
_____
_____
_____
_____

Diary

Date _____

_____
_____
_____
_____
_____

Date _____

_____
_____
_____
_____
_____

Date _____

_____
_____
_____
_____
_____

Date _____

_____
_____
_____
_____
_____

Date _____

_____
_____
_____
_____
_____

Diary

Date _____

_____
_____
_____
_____
_____
_____

Date _____

_____
_____
_____
_____
_____
_____

Date _____

_____
_____
_____
_____
_____
_____

Date _____

_____
_____
_____
_____
_____
_____

Date _____

_____
_____
_____
_____
_____
_____

Diary

Date _____

_____
_____
_____
_____
_____

Date _____

_____
_____
_____
_____
_____
_____

Date _____

_____
_____
_____
_____
_____
_____

Date _____

_____
_____
_____
_____
_____

Date _____

_____
_____
_____
_____
_____

Diary

Date _____

_____
_____
_____
_____
_____
_____

Date _____

_____
_____
_____
_____
_____
_____

Date _____

_____
_____
_____
_____
_____
_____

Date _____

_____
_____
_____
_____
_____

Date _____

_____
_____
_____
_____
_____
_____

Diary

Date _____

_____
_____
_____
_____
_____

Date _____

_____
_____
_____
_____
_____

Date _____

_____
_____
_____
_____
_____

Date _____

_____
_____
_____
_____

Date _____

_____
_____
_____
_____

Diary

Date _____

_____
_____
_____
_____
_____

Date _____

_____
_____
_____
_____
_____
_____

Date _____

_____
_____
_____
_____
_____
_____

Date _____

_____
_____
_____
_____
_____

Date _____

_____
_____
_____
_____
_____

Diary

Date _____

Date _____

Date _____

Date _____

Date _____

Diary

Date _____

_____
_____
_____
_____
_____

Date _____

_____
_____
_____
_____
_____

Date _____

_____
_____
_____
_____
_____

Date _____

_____
_____
_____
_____
_____

Date _____

_____
_____
_____
_____
_____

Diary

Date _____

_____
_____
_____
_____
_____
_____

Date _____

_____
_____
_____
_____
_____
_____

Date _____

_____
_____
_____
_____
_____
_____

Date _____

_____
_____
_____
_____
_____
_____

Date _____

_____
_____
_____
_____
_____
_____

Diary

Date _____

_____
_____
_____
_____
_____

Date _____

_____
_____
_____
_____
_____

Date _____

_____
_____
_____
_____
_____

Date _____

_____
_____
_____
_____
_____

Date _____

_____
_____
_____
_____
_____

Diary

Date _____

_____
_____
_____
_____
_____
_____

Date _____

_____
_____
_____
_____
_____
_____

Date _____

_____
_____
_____
_____
_____
_____

Date _____

_____
_____
_____
_____

Date _____

_____
_____
_____
_____

Diary

Date _____

_____
_____
_____
_____
_____

Date _____

_____
_____
_____
_____
_____
_____

Date _____

_____
_____
_____
_____
_____
_____

Date _____

_____
_____
_____
_____
_____
_____

Date _____

_____
_____
_____
_____
_____
_____

Diary

Date _____

_____
_____
_____
_____
_____

Date _____

_____
_____
_____
_____
_____

Date _____

_____
_____
_____
_____
_____

Date _____

_____
_____
_____
_____
_____

Date _____

_____
_____
_____
_____
_____

Diary

Date _____

_____
_____
_____
_____
_____

Date _____

_____
_____
_____
_____
_____

Date _____

_____
_____
_____
_____
_____

Date _____

_____
_____
_____
_____
_____

Date _____

_____
_____
_____
_____
_____

Diary

Date _____

_____
_____
_____
_____
_____
_____

Date _____

_____
_____
_____
_____
_____
_____

Date _____

_____
_____
_____
_____
_____
_____

Date _____

_____
_____
_____
_____
_____
_____

Date _____

_____
_____
_____
_____
_____
_____

Diary

Date _____

_____
_____
_____
_____
_____
_____

Date _____

_____
_____
_____
_____
_____
_____

Date _____

_____
_____
_____
_____
_____
_____

Date _____

_____
_____
_____
_____
_____

Date _____

_____
_____
_____
_____
_____

Diary

Date _____

_____
_____
_____
_____
_____

Date _____

_____
_____
_____
_____
_____

Date _____

_____
_____
_____
_____
_____

Date _____

_____
_____
_____
_____

Date _____

_____
_____
_____
_____

Diary

Date _____

_____
_____
_____
_____
_____

Date _____

_____
_____
_____
_____
_____
_____

Date _____

_____
_____
_____
_____
_____
_____

Date _____

_____
_____
_____
_____
_____

Date _____

_____
_____
_____
_____
_____

Diary

Date _____

_____
_____
_____
_____
_____

Date _____

_____
_____
_____
_____
_____
_____

Date _____

_____
_____
_____
_____
_____
_____

Date _____

_____
_____
_____
_____
_____

Date _____

_____
_____
_____
_____
_____

Diary

Date _____

_____
_____
_____
_____
_____

Date _____

_____
_____
_____
_____
_____

Date _____

_____
_____
_____
_____
_____

Date _____

_____
_____
_____
_____

Date _____

_____
_____
_____
_____

Diary

Date _____

_____
_____
_____
_____
_____
_____

Date _____

_____
_____
_____
_____
_____
_____

Date _____

_____
_____
_____
_____
_____
_____

Date _____

_____
_____
_____
_____
_____

Date _____

_____
_____
_____
_____
_____

Diary

Date _____

_____
_____
_____
_____
_____

Date _____

_____
_____
_____
_____
_____

Date _____

_____
_____
_____
_____
_____

Date _____

_____
_____
_____
_____

Date _____

_____
_____
_____
_____
_____

Diary

Date _____

_____
_____
_____
_____
_____
_____

Date _____

_____
_____
_____
_____
_____
_____

Date _____

_____
_____
_____
_____
_____
_____

Date _____

_____
_____
_____
_____
_____

Date _____

_____
_____
_____
_____
_____

Diary

Date _____

_____
_____
_____
_____
_____
_____

Date _____

_____
_____
_____
_____
_____
_____

Date _____

_____
_____
_____
_____
_____
_____

Date _____

_____
_____
_____
_____
_____

Date _____

_____
_____
_____
_____
_____

Diary

Date _____

_____
_____
_____
_____
_____
_____

Date _____

_____
_____
_____
_____
_____
_____

Date _____

_____
_____
_____
_____
_____
_____

Date _____

_____
_____
_____
_____
_____
_____

Date _____

_____
_____
_____
_____
_____
_____

Diary

Date _____

_____
_____
_____
_____
_____
_____

Date _____

_____
_____
_____
_____
_____
_____

Date _____

_____
_____
_____
_____
_____
_____

Date _____

_____
_____
_____
_____

Date _____

_____
_____
_____
_____
_____

Diary

Date _____

_____
_____
_____
_____
_____

Date _____

_____
_____
_____
_____
_____

Date _____

_____
_____
_____
_____
_____

Date _____

_____
_____
_____
_____
_____

Date _____

_____
_____
_____
_____
_____

Diary

Date _____

_____
_____
_____
_____
_____

Date _____

_____
_____
_____
_____
_____

Date _____

_____
_____
_____
_____
_____

Date _____

_____
_____
_____
_____
_____

Date _____

_____
_____
_____
_____
_____

Diary

Date _____

_____
_____
_____
_____
_____

Date _____

_____
_____
_____
_____
_____

Date _____

_____
_____
_____
_____
_____

Date _____

_____
_____
_____
_____
_____

Date _____

_____
_____
_____
_____
_____

Diary

Date _____

_____
_____
_____
_____
_____
_____

Date _____

_____
_____
_____
_____
_____
_____

Date _____

_____
_____
_____
_____
_____
_____

Date _____

_____
_____
_____
_____
_____
_____

Date _____

_____
_____
_____
_____
_____
_____

Diary

Date _____

_____
_____
_____
_____
_____

Date _____

_____
_____
_____
_____
_____

Date _____

_____
_____
_____
_____
_____

Date _____

_____
_____
_____
_____

Date _____

_____
_____
_____
_____

Diary

Date _____

_____
_____
_____
_____
_____

Date _____

_____
_____
_____
_____
_____

Date _____

_____
_____
_____
_____
_____

Date _____

_____
_____
_____
_____

Date _____

_____
_____
_____
_____

Diary

Date _____

_____
_____
_____
_____
_____
_____

Date _____

_____
_____
_____
_____
_____
_____

Date _____

_____
_____
_____
_____
_____
_____

Date _____

_____
_____
_____
_____
_____

Date _____

_____
_____
_____
_____
_____

Diary

Date _____

_____
_____
_____
_____
_____

Date _____

_____
_____
_____
_____
_____
_____

Date _____

_____
_____
_____
_____
_____
_____

Date _____

_____
_____
_____
_____
_____

Date _____

_____
_____
_____
_____
_____

Diary

Date _____

_____
_____
_____
_____
_____

Date _____

_____
_____
_____
_____
_____

Date _____

_____
_____
_____
_____
_____

Date _____

_____
_____
_____
_____
_____

Date _____

_____
_____
_____
_____
_____

Diary

Date _____

_____
_____
_____
_____
_____

Date _____

_____
_____
_____
_____
_____

Date _____

_____
_____
_____
_____
_____

Date _____

_____
_____
_____
_____
_____

Date _____

_____
_____
_____
_____
_____

Diary

Date _____

_____
_____
_____
_____
_____
_____

Date _____

_____
_____
_____
_____
_____
_____

Date _____

_____
_____
_____
_____
_____
_____

Date _____

_____
_____
_____
_____
_____
_____

Date _____

_____
_____
_____
_____
_____
_____

Diary

Date _____

_____
_____
_____
_____
_____

Date _____

_____
_____
_____
_____
_____

Date _____

_____
_____
_____
_____
_____

Date _____

_____
_____
_____
_____
_____

Date _____

_____
_____
_____
_____
_____

Notes

Section 11

Notes

Writing down any and all thoughts came in handy for the times when we just couldn't remember everything.

For instance:

- Type of treatment chosen, and why.

- Things to discuss with In-Home Health Services.

- Names of individuals who went out of their way to help. (When further assistance was needed, we requested that same person).

- A list of what to pack and take to the hospital. Mom usually had a bag ready to go so she wouldn't forget anything.

- Errands Mom needed someone to do for her.

- Dates, names and places to call for getting test results.

- Making arrangements for appointments and other outings.

- Latest information regarding an illness and its source; i.e., newspaper article, radio/TV discussion, etc.

- A list of what bills to pay and when.

Notes

Notes

Notes

Notes

Notes

Notes

Notes

Notes

Notes

Notes

Messages

Section 12

Messages

During Mom's illness, there were times we took turns staying with her throughout the day, on weekends and during the week. There was also a period of time when Mom went to live with family members. Sometimes we wrote down questions, comments, notes for follow-up and items of importance, regarding Mom. When changing shifts, some messages required discussion.

This reference made it easy for the next caregiver to takeover and pickup where the previous caregiver left off. Leaving messages was a good way to communicate between each other without disturbing her.

The following is one of our messages:

Mom's leg hurt today. Placed a call to the doctor. Prescription refill was called in and will be ready later today. I'll pick it up when I go to the grocery store, tonight. Can you think of anything Mom needs? She ate two good meals today. At breakfast Mom had one slice of toast, a little bit of scrambled egg, a few bites of banana and an a protein drink. She slept through lunch. Later, about 1:30 she wanted to get up and eat. She had a small bowl of soup, a cracker and a few sips of soda. Uncle Lyle called today, while Mom was asleep. Doctor called back...wants to see Mom. Can you take her there, on Thursday? Would you call and make a appointment? If you're not available, I can take her. Home Health came this morning and bathed Mom. We changed the sheets. Notice the new arrangement of medications on the night stand. I think it will be easier to have them lined up by name, with the time the next dose should be given. This way the next dose is ready ahead of time. I'm going to be in a meeting all day tomorrow; page me if you need me.

Messages and Correspondence from Caregiver to Caregiver

By: _____ **Date:** _____

_____
_____
_____
_____
_____
_____

By: _____ **Date:** _____

_____
_____
_____
_____
_____
_____

By: _____ **Date:** _____

_____
_____
_____
_____
_____
_____

By: _____ **Date:** _____

_____
_____
_____
_____

By: _____ **Date:** _____

_____
_____
_____
_____
_____

Messages and Correspondence from Caregiver to Caregiver

By: _____ **Date:** _____

_____
_____
_____
_____
_____

By: _____ **Date:** _____

_____
_____
_____
_____
_____
_____

By: _____ **Date:** _____

_____
_____
_____
_____
_____

By: _____ **Date:** _____

_____
_____
_____
_____

By: _____ **Date:** _____

_____
_____
_____
_____

Messages and Correspondence from Caregiver to Caregiver

By: _____ **Date:** _____

_____
_____
_____
_____
_____
_____

By: _____ **Date:** _____

_____
_____
_____
_____
_____
_____

By: _____ **Date:** _____

_____
_____
_____
_____
_____
_____

By: _____ **Date:** _____

_____
_____
_____
_____
_____

By: _____ **Date:** _____

_____
_____
_____
_____
_____

Messages and Correspondence from Caregiver to Caregiver

By: _____ **Date:** _____

_____
_____
_____
_____
_____

By: _____ **Date:** _____

_____
_____
_____
_____
_____

By: _____ **Date:** _____

_____
_____
_____
_____
_____

By: _____ **Date:** _____

_____
_____
_____
_____
_____

By: _____ **Date:** _____

_____
_____
_____
_____
_____

Messages and Correspondence from Caregiver to Caregiver

By: _____ **Date:** _____
_____
_____
_____
_____
_____
_____

By: _____ **Date:** _____
_____
_____
_____
_____
_____
_____

By: _____ **Date:** _____
_____
_____
_____
_____
_____
_____

By: _____ **Date:** _____
_____
_____
_____
_____
_____

By: _____ **Date:** _____
_____
_____
_____
_____
_____

Messages and Correspondence from Caregiver to Caregiver

By: _____ **Date:** _____
_____
_____
_____
_____
_____

By: _____ **Date:** _____
_____
_____
_____
_____
_____

By: _____ **Date:** _____
_____
_____
_____
_____
_____

By: _____ **Date:** _____
_____
_____
_____
_____
_____

By: _____ **Date:** _____
_____
_____
_____
_____
_____

Messages and Correspondence from Caregiver to Caregiver

By: _____ Date: _____

_____
_____
_____
_____
_____

By: _____ Date: _____

_____
_____
_____
_____
_____
_____

By: _____ Date: _____

_____
_____
_____
_____
_____
_____

By: _____ Date: _____

_____
_____
_____
_____

By: _____ Date: _____

_____
_____
_____
_____
_____

Messages and Correspondence from Caregiver to Caregiver

By: _____   **Date:** _____
_____
_____
_____
_____
_____

By: _____   **Date:** _____
_____
_____
_____
_____
_____

By: _____   **Date:** _____
_____
_____
_____
_____
_____

By: _____   **Date:** _____
_____
_____
_____
_____
_____

By: _____   **Date:** _____
_____
_____
_____
_____
_____

Messages and Correspondence from Caregiver to Caregiver

By: _____ **Date:** _____
_____
_____
_____
_____
_____
_____

By: _____ **Date:** _____
_____
_____
_____
_____
_____
_____

By: _____ **Date:** _____
_____
_____
_____
_____
_____
_____

By: _____ **Date:** _____
_____
_____
_____
_____
_____

By: _____ **Date:** _____
_____
_____
_____
_____
_____

Messages and Correspondence from Caregiver to Caregiver

By: _____ **Date:** _____

_____
_____
_____
_____
_____

By: _____ **Date:** _____

_____
_____
_____
_____
_____

By: _____ **Date:** _____

_____
_____
_____
_____
_____

By: _____ **Date:** _____

_____
_____
_____
_____

By: _____ **Date:** _____

_____
_____
_____
_____

Messages and Correspondence from Caregiver to Caregiver

By: _____ **Date:** _____
_____
_____
_____
_____
_____

By: _____ **Date:** _____
_____
_____
_____
_____
_____

By: _____ **Date:** _____
_____
_____
_____
_____
_____

By: _____ **Date:** _____
_____
_____
_____
_____
_____

By: _____ **Date:** _____
_____
_____
_____
_____
_____

Messages and Correspondence from Caregiver to Caregiver

By: _____   Date: _____

_____
_____
_____
_____
_____
_____

By: _____   Date: _____

_____
_____
_____
_____
_____
_____

By: _____   Date: _____

_____
_____
_____
_____
_____
_____

By: _____   Date: _____

_____
_____
_____
_____
_____

By: _____   Date: _____

_____
_____
_____
_____
_____
_____

Messages and Correspondence from Caregiver to Caregiver

By: _____ **Date:** _____
_____
_____
_____
_____
_____
_____

By: _____ **Date:** _____
_____
_____
_____
_____
_____
_____

By: _____ **Date:** _____
_____
_____
_____
_____
_____
_____

By: _____ **Date:** _____
_____
_____
_____
_____
_____

By: _____ **Date:** _____
_____
_____
_____
_____
_____

Messages and Correspondence from Caregiver to Caregiver

By: _____ Date: _____

_____
_____
_____
_____
_____

By: _____ Date: _____

_____
_____
_____
_____
_____

By: _____ Date: _____

_____
_____
_____
_____
_____

By: _____ Date: _____

_____
_____
_____
_____
_____

By: _____ Date: _____

_____
_____
_____
_____
_____

Messages and Correspondence from Caregiver to Caregiver

By: _____ **Date:** _____

_____
_____
_____
_____
_____

By: _____ **Date:** _____

_____
_____
_____
_____
_____

By: _____ **Date:** _____

_____
_____
_____
_____
_____

By: _____ **Date:** _____

_____
_____
_____
_____
_____

By: _____ **Date:** _____

_____
_____
_____
_____

Messages and Correspondence from Caregiver to Caregiver

By: _____ **Date:** _____

_____
_____
_____
_____
_____

By: _____ **Date:** _____

_____
_____
_____
_____
_____
_____

By: _____ **Date:** _____

_____
_____
_____
_____
_____
_____

By: _____ **Date:** _____

_____
_____
_____
_____
_____

By: _____ **Date:** _____

_____
_____
_____
_____
_____

Messages and Correspondence from Caregiver to Caregiver

By: _____ **Date:** _____

_____
_____
_____
_____
_____

By: _____ **Date:** _____

_____
_____
_____
_____
_____
_____

By: _____ **Date:** _____

_____
_____
_____
_____
_____
_____

By: _____ **Date:** _____

_____
_____
_____
_____
_____

By: _____ **Date:** _____

_____
_____
_____
_____
_____

Messages and Correspondence from Caregiver to Caregiver

By: _____ **Date:** _____

_____
_____
_____
_____
_____
_____

By: _____ **Date:** _____

_____
_____
_____
_____
_____
_____

By: _____ **Date:** _____

_____
_____
_____
_____
_____
_____

By: _____ **Date:** _____

_____
_____
_____
_____
_____

By: _____ **Date:** _____

_____
_____
_____
_____
_____

Messages and Correspondence from Caregiver to Caregiver

By: _____ **Date:** _____

_____
_____
_____
_____
_____
_____

By: _____ **Date:** _____

_____
_____
_____
_____
_____
_____

By: _____ **Date:** _____

_____
_____
_____
_____
_____
_____

By: _____ **Date:** _____

_____
_____
_____
_____
_____

By: _____ **Date:** _____

_____
_____
_____
_____
_____
_____

Messages and Correspondence from Caregiver to Caregiver

By: _____ **Date:** _____

_____
_____
_____
_____
_____

By: _____ **Date:** _____

_____
_____
_____
_____
_____
_____

By: _____ **Date:** _____

_____
_____
_____
_____
_____
_____

By: _____ **Date:** _____

_____
_____
_____
_____

By: _____ **Date:** _____

_____
_____
_____
_____
_____

Miscellaneous

Section 13

Miscellaneous

This section is designed for any extra items we saved to have readily available.

To help keep items in one accessible location, either tape them to blank pages or use some type of file folder...storage of copies, which might include signed documents...etc.

Miscellaneous Items

Miscellaneous Items

Comments and Suggestions

Section 14

Comments, and Suggestions

In order to update this book to help meet your needs, please send comments and suggestions to:

HopeWorks Medical Diary
P.O. Box 754
Los Alamitos, CA 90720-0754

Order Form for
HopeWorks Medical Diary...A Patient's Daily Log

Name: _____

Street: _____

City/State/Zip: _____

Hm Phone: (_ _ _) _ _ _ - _ _ _ _   Wk Phone: (_ _ _) _ _ _ - _ _ _ _

Qty	Amount	Total
_____	$24.95 each book	_____
	California Residents add 7.75% sales tax	_____
	Shipping and Handling $5.95	
	Add $2.50 for each additional book shipped to same address	_____
	Total	_____

Send Check or Money Order to:

HopeWorks
P.O. Box 754, Los Alamitos, CA 90720-0754

As we work together for those in need

HopeWorks Medical Diary
A Patient's Daily Log

can be ordered in large quantities for
Association's, Foundation's, Societies, Bookstores, Clinic's, Hospitals,
HMO's, PPO's, Insurance Companies, Senior Citizen Plans, Pharmacies...etc.

Please send request on letterhead to:
HopeWorks, P.O. Box 754, Los Alamitos, CA 90720-0754

Copyright by Donna L. Hope 1996. All Rights Reserved Worldwide.

Order Form for HopeWorks Permanent Record Booklet

Name: _____

Street: _____

City/State/Zip: _____

Hm Phone: (___) ___-____   Wk Phone: (___) ___-____

The HopeWorks Permanent Record Booklet is designed to conveniently fit into a small safe deposit box. Storing the following information will be helpful in case of emergency, disaster or death.

Booklet includes:

Emergency Telephone Numbers and Addresses, Safe Deposit Box Suggestions, Financial Guide, Inventory of Household Belongings, Personal History, Funeral Arrangement Information, Comments/Suggestions.

Qty	Amount	Total
_____	$7.95 each book...........................	_____
	California Residents add 7.75% sales tax......	_____
	Shipping and Handling per each booklet......	$1.00
	Total	_____

Send Check or Money Order to:

HopeWorks
P.O. Box 754
Los Alamitos, CA 90720-0754

What's Mom doing up there?

It's Thanksgiving morning and I'm in the kitchen preparing a feast for another family holiday.

As I place the pies in the oven, I realize--*this is our first Christmas without Mother*...here.

This holiday season will be different than any I've ever experienced before...Mom won't be with us.

She died in April, after a two year battle with cancer.

Nothing can replace the absence of Mom at the Thanksgiving table, or opening gifts Christmas morning.

Christmas Eve was Mom's favorite time to entertain with family and friends at her place after church service.

Even as we continue attending church service through the years on Christmas Eve, she won't be here, to serve another one of her delicious dinners, followed by games and laughter.

I can't help wonder--*what's she doing up there?*

I imagine Heaven to be filled with angels singing and playing musical instruments to honor our King...

>BUT, are they baking delicious turkeys?

>And is Mom preparing her famous gravy?

>And who will play our favorite family games with Mom?

>Do they have chairs to fall off of when they laugh really hard like we do?

Preparing this great meal isn't so fun anymore.

Later that morning when the food was ready, and my family was waiting for our guests to arrive, I felt a peace come over me.

How excited I became when I realized, it was not intended to be our first holiday without Mother...but **her first Christmas celebration with our dear Lord and Savior!**

How special Mom must be, for the Lord to have called her to His Mansion to celebrate it with Him.

In a few days it will be time to decorate for Christmas.

All the stockings will hang in their usual places on the fireplace, including Mothers.

Only, hers will already be filled...with a lovely Angel doll, dressed in white, with sparkly silver wings and a cute halo on top of the curly brunette hair.

The Angel is holding a wrapped gift, reaching out as if she is handing the gift to anyone that passes by.

It is Mom's gift to us...her family and friends--memories of the love we shared while we were on earth together.

When we open our gifts Christmas morning, my thoughts will be with Mom. I will picture the angels stop singing and playing music, for a time of quietness, while Jesus, Himself, sits with Mother and all the others, telling the complete story of the Miracle Birth, God sent to us so long ago.

Even though we are filled with emptiness in the loss of Mom, she has already begun her new journey into eternity...a new beginning that will continue through all the seasons in Heaven.

How fortunate we are, to belong to the family of God, saved by His grace that, someday, we will again sit with Mom, as we celebrate together, hearing first hand the blessed story from the King of Kings ♥

Donna L. Hope
November 1996